100 CALORIE DIET
TRACK YOUR WEIGHT LOSS PROGRESS

Copyright 2015

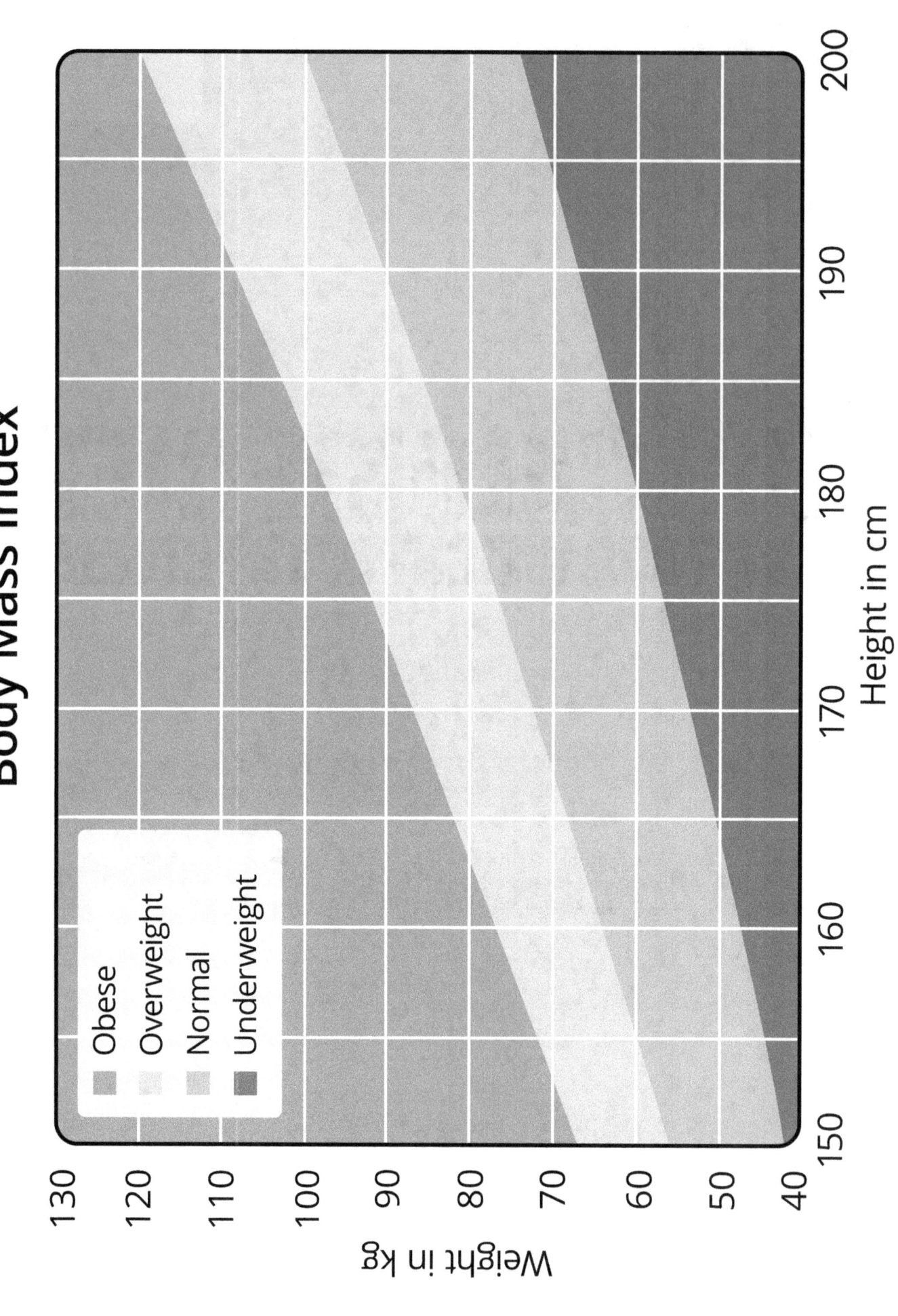

WEIGHT CATEGORIES

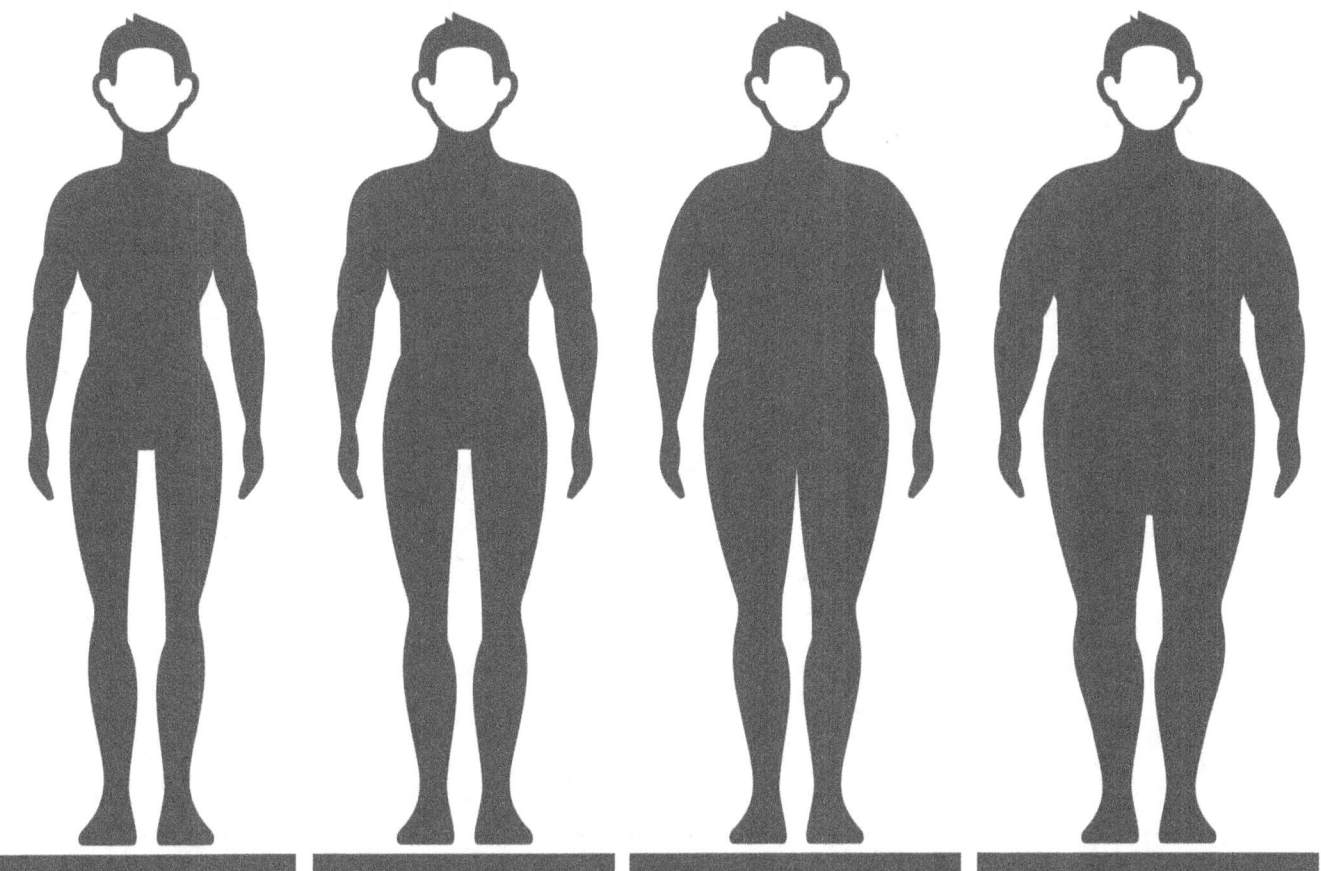

UNDERWEIGHT	HEALTHY	OVERWEIGHT	OBESE
< 18.5	18.5-24.9	25.0-29.9	> 30.0

Adult BMI Calculation Formula

$$\text{BMI} = \frac{(\textbf{your weight} \text{ in pounds}) \times 703}{(\textbf{your height} \text{ in inches})^2}$$

PERSONAL GOALS

Start Date: _____ End Date: _____

My Goals: _____

_____

_____

My Plans: _____

_____

_____

Daily Food Targets

calories	fat	carbs	fiber

protein	_____	_____	(dashed box)

My Statistics

GOAL	RECORD ONE OR MORE	BEFORE	AFTER	NET +/-
	weight			
	cholesterol level			
	blood pressure			
	MEASUREMENTS:			
	chest			
	waist			
	hip			
	neck			
	upper arms			
	thighs			
	calves			

Before Pictures Here

After Pictures Here

FOOD	QTY	CALS	CARBS	PROTEIN (g)	FAT (g)
BREAKFAST					
Sub Total					
LUNCH					
Sub Total					
DINNER					
Sub Total					
SNACK					
Sub Total					
Total					

NUTRIENT	TOTAL	UNITS	GOAL %	RDA%
Calories				
Fat				
Saturated Fat				
Polyunsaturated				
Monounsaturated				

FOOD	QTY	CALS	CARBS	PROTEIN (g)	FAT (g)
BREAKFAST					
Sub Total					
LUNCH					
Sub Total					
DINNER					
Sub Total					
SNACK					
Sub Total					
Total					

NUTRIENT	TOTAL	UNITS	GOAL %	RDA%
Calories				
Fat				
Saturated Fat				
Polyunsaturated				
Monounsaturated				

FOOD	QTY	CALS	CARBS	PROTEIN (g)	FAT (g)
BREAKFAST					
Sub Total					
LUNCH					
Sub Total					
DINNER					
Sub Total					
SNACK					
Sub Total					
Total					

NUTRIENT	TOTAL	UNITS	GOAL %	RDA%
Calories				
Fat				
Saturated Fat				
Polyunsaturated				
Monounsaturated				

FOOD	QTY	CALS	CARBS	PROTEIN (g)	FAT (g)
BREAKFAST					
Sub Total					
LUNCH					
Sub Total					
DINNER					
Sub Total					
SNACK					
Sub Total					
Total					

NUTRIENT	TOTAL	UNITS	GOAL %	RDA%
Calories				
Fat				
Saturated Fat				
Polyunsaturated				
Monounsaturated				

FOOD		QTY	CALS	CARBS	PROTEIN (g)	FAT (g)
BREAKFAST						
	Sub Total					
LUNCH						
	Sub Total					
DINNER						
	Sub Total					
SNACK						
	Sub Total					
	Total					

NUTRIENT	TOTAL	UNITS	GOAL %	RDA%
Calories				
Fat				
Saturated Fat				
Polyunsaturated				
Monounsaturated				

FOOD	QTY	CALS	CARBS	PROTEIN (g)	FAT (g)
BREAKFAST					
Sub Total					
LUNCH					
Sub Total					
DINNER					
Sub Total					
SNACK					
Sub Total					
Total					

NUTRIENT	TOTAL	UNITS	GOAL %	RDA%
Calories				
Fat				
Saturated Fat				
Polyunsaturated				
Monounsaturated				

FOOD	QTY	CALS	CARBS	PROTEIN (g)	FAT (g)
BREAKFAST					
Sub Total					
LUNCH					
Sub Total					
DINNER					
Sub Total					
SNACK					
Sub Total					
Total					

NUTRIENT	TOTAL	UNITS	GOAL %	RDA%
Calories				
Fat				
Saturated Fat				
Polyunsaturated				
Monounsaturated				

FOOD	QTY	CALS	CARBS	PROTEIN (g)	FAT (g)
BREAKFAST					
Sub Total					
LUNCH					
Sub Total					
DINNER					
Sub Total					
SNACK					
Sub Total					
Total					

NUTRIENT	TOTAL	UNITS	GOAL %	RDA%
Calories				
Fat				
Saturated Fat				
Polyunsaturated				
Monounsaturated				

FOOD	QTY	CALS	CARBS	PROTEIN (g)	FAT (g)
BREAKFAST					
Sub Total					
LUNCH					
Sub Total					
DINNER					
Sub Total					
SNACK					
Sub Total					
Total					

NUTRIENT	TOTAL	UNITS	GOAL %	RDA%
Calories				
Fat				
Saturated Fat				
Polyunsaturated				
Monounsaturated				

FOOD	QTY	CALS	CARBS	PROTEIN (g)	FAT (g)
BREAKFAST					
Sub Total					
LUNCH					
Sub Total					
DINNER					
Sub Total					
SNACK					
Sub Total					
Total					

NUTRIENT	TOTAL	UNITS	GOAL %	RDA%
Calories				
Fat				
Saturated Fat				
Polyunsaturated				
Monounsaturated				

FOOD	QTY	CALS	CARBS	PROTEIN (g)	FAT (g)
BREAKFAST					
Sub Total					
LUNCH					
Sub Total					
DINNER					
Sub Total					
SNACK					
Sub Total					
Total					

NUTRIENT	TOTAL	UNITS	GOAL %	RDA%
Calories				
Fat				
Saturated Fat				
Polyunsaturated				
Monounsaturated				

FOOD	QTY	CALS	CARBS	PROTEIN (g)	FAT (g)
BREAKFAST					
Sub Total					
LUNCH					
Sub Total					
DINNER					
Sub Total					
SNACK					
Sub Total					
Total					

NUTRIENT	TOTAL	UNITS	GOAL %	RDA%
Calories				
Fat				
Saturated Fat				
Polyunsaturated				
Monounsaturated				

FOOD	QTY	CALS	CARBS	PROTEIN (g)	FAT (g)
BREAKFAST					
Sub Total					
LUNCH					
Sub Total					
DINNER					
Sub Total					
SNACK					
Sub Total					
Total					

NUTRIENT	TOTAL	UNITS	GOAL %	RDA%
Calories				
Fat				
Saturated Fat				
Polyunsaturated				
Monounsaturated				

FOOD	QTY	CALS	CARBS	PROTEIN (g)	FAT (g)
BREAKFAST					
Sub Total					
LUNCH					
Sub Total					
DINNER					
Sub Total					
SNACK					
Sub Total					
Total					

NUTRIENT	TOTAL	UNITS	GOAL %	RDA%
Calories				
Fat				
Saturated Fat				
Polyunsaturated				
Monounsaturated				

FOOD	QTY	CALS	CARBS	PROTEIN (g)	FAT (g)
BREAKFAST					
Sub Total					
LUNCH					
Sub Total					
DINNER					
Sub Total					
SNACK					
Sub Total					
Total					

NUTRIENT	TOTAL	UNITS	GOAL %	RDA%
Calories				
Fat				
Saturated Fat				
Polyunsaturated				
Monounsaturated				

FOOD	QTY	CALS	CARBS	PROTEIN (g)	FAT (g)
BREAKFAST					
Sub Total					
LUNCH					
Sub Total					
DINNER					
Sub Total					
SNACK					
Sub Total					
Total					

NUTRIENT	TOTAL	UNITS	GOAL %	RDA%
Calories				
Fat				
Saturated Fat				
Polyunsaturated				
Monounsaturated				

FOOD	QTY	CALS	CARBS	PROTEIN (g)	FAT (g)
BREAKFAST					
Sub Total					
LUNCH					
Sub Total					
DINNER					
Sub Total					
SNACK					
Sub Total					
Total					

NUTRIENT	TOTAL	UNITS	GOAL %	RDA%
Calories				
Fat				
Saturated Fat				
Polyunsaturated				
Monounsaturated				

FOOD	QTY	CALS	CARBS	PROTEIN (g)	FAT (g)
BREAKFAST					
Sub Total					
LUNCH					
Sub Total					
DINNER					
Sub Total					
SNACK					
Sub Total					
Total					

NUTRIENT	TOTAL	UNITS	GOAL %	RDA%
Calories				
Fat				
Saturated Fat				
Polyunsaturated				
Monounsaturated				

FOOD	QTY	CALS	CARBS	PROTEIN (g)	FAT (g)
BREAKFAST					
Sub Total					
LUNCH					
Sub Total					
DINNER					
Sub Total					
SNACK					
Sub Total					
Total					

NUTRIENT	TOTAL	UNITS	GOAL %	RDA%
Calories				
Fat				
Saturated Fat				
Polyunsaturated				
Monounsaturated				

FOOD	QTY	CALS	CARBS	PROTEIN (g)	FAT (g)
BREAKFAST					
Sub Total					
LUNCH					
Sub Total					
DINNER					
Sub Total					
SNACK					
Sub Total					
Total					

NUTRIENT	TOTAL	UNITS	GOAL %	RDA%
Calories				
Fat				
Saturated Fat				
Polyunsaturated				
Monounsaturated				

FOOD	QTY	CALS	CARBS	PROTEIN (g)	FAT (g)
BREAKFAST					
Sub Total					
LUNCH					
Sub Total					
DINNER					
Sub Total					
SNACK					
Sub Total					
Total					

NUTRIENT	TOTAL	UNITS	GOAL %	RDA%
Calories				
Fat				
Saturated Fat				
Polyunsaturated				
Monounsaturated				

FOOD	QTY	CALS	CARBS	PROTEIN (g)	FAT (g)
BREAKFAST					
Sub Total					
LUNCH					
Sub Total					
DINNER					
Sub Total					
SNACK					
Sub Total					
Total					

NUTRIENT	TOTAL	UNITS	GOAL %	RDA%
Calories				
Fat				
Saturated Fat				
Polyunsaturated				
Monounsaturated				

FOOD	QTY	CALS	CARBS	PROTEIN (g)	FAT (g)
BREAKFAST					
Sub Total					
LUNCH					
Sub Total					
DINNER					
Sub Total					
SNACK					
Sub Total					
Total					

NUTRIENT	TOTAL	UNITS	GOAL %	RDA%
Calories				
Fat				
Saturated Fat				
Polyunsaturated				
Monounsaturated				

FOOD	QTY	CALS	CARBS	PROTEIN (g)	FAT (g)
BREAKFAST					
Sub Total					
LUNCH					
Sub Total					
DINNER					
Sub Total					
SNACK					
Sub Total					
Total					

NUTRIENT	TOTAL	UNITS	GOAL %	RDA%
Calories				
Fat				
Saturated Fat				
Polyunsaturated				
Monounsaturated				

FOOD	QTY	CALS	CARBS	PROTEIN (g)	FAT (g)
BREAKFAST					
Sub Total					
LUNCH					
Sub Total					
DINNER					
Sub Total					
SNACK					
Sub Total					
Total					

NUTRIENT	TOTAL	UNITS	GOAL %	RDA%
Calories				
Fat				
Saturated Fat				
Polyunsaturated				
Monounsaturated				

FOOD	QTY	CALS	CARBS	PROTEIN (g)	FAT (g)
BREAKFAST					
Sub Total					
LUNCH					
Sub Total					
DINNER					
Sub Total					
SNACK					
Sub Total					
Total					

NUTRIENT	TOTAL	UNITS	GOAL %	RDA%
Calories				
Fat				
Saturated Fat				
Polyunsaturated				
Monounsaturated				

FOOD	QTY	CALS	CARBS	PROTEIN (g)	FAT (g)
BREAKFAST					
Sub Total					
LUNCH					
Sub Total					
DINNER					
Sub Total					
SNACK					
Sub Total					
Total					

NUTRIENT	TOTAL	UNITS	GOAL %	RDA%
Calories				
Fat				
Saturated Fat				
Polyunsaturated				
Monounsaturated				

FOOD	QTY	CALS	CARBS	PROTEIN (g)	FAT (g)
BREAKFAST					
Sub Total					
LUNCH					
Sub Total					
DINNER					
Sub Total					
SNACK					
Sub Total					
Total					

NUTRIENT	TOTAL	UNITS	GOAL %	RDA%
Calories				
Fat				
Saturated Fat				
Polyunsaturated				
Monounsaturated				

FOOD	QTY	CALS	CARBS	PROTEIN (g)	FAT (g)
BREAKFAST					
Sub Total					
LUNCH					
Sub Total					
DINNER					
Sub Total					
SNACK					
Sub Total					
Total					

NUTRIENT	TOTAL	UNITS	GOAL %	RDA%
Calories				
Fat				
Saturated Fat				
Polyunsaturated				
Monounsaturated				

FOOD	QTY	CALS	CARBS	PROTEIN (g)	FAT (g)
BREAKFAST					
Sub Total					
LUNCH					
Sub Total					
DINNER					
Sub Total					
SNACK					
Sub Total					
Total					

NUTRIENT	TOTAL	UNITS	GOAL %	RDA%
Calories				
Fat				
Saturated Fat				
Polyunsaturated				
Monounsaturated				

FOOD	QTY	CALS	CARBS	PROTEIN (g)	FAT (g)
BREAKFAST					
Sub Total					
LUNCH					
Sub Total					
DINNER					
Sub Total					
SNACK					
Sub Total					
Total					

NUTRIENT	TOTAL	UNITS	GOAL %	RDA%
Calories				
Fat				
Saturated Fat				
Polyunsaturated				
Monounsaturated				

FOOD	QTY	CALS	CARBS	PROTEIN (g)	FAT (g)
BREAKFAST					
Sub Total					
LUNCH					
Sub Total					
DINNER					
Sub Total					
SNACK					
Sub Total					
Total					

NUTRIENT	TOTAL	UNITS	GOAL %	RDA%
Calories				
Fat				
Saturated Fat				
Polyunsaturated				
Monounsaturated				

FOOD	QTY	CALS	CARBS	PROTEIN (g)	FAT (g)
BREAKFAST					
Sub Total					
LUNCH					
Sub Total					
DINNER					
Sub Total					
SNACK					
Sub Total					
Total					

NUTRIENT	TOTAL	UNITS	GOAL %	RDA%
Calories				
Fat				
Saturated Fat				
Polyunsaturated				
Monounsaturated				

FOOD	QTY	CALS	CARBS	PROTEIN (g)	FAT (g)
BREAKFAST					
Sub Total					
LUNCH					
Sub Total					
DINNER					
Sub Total					
SNACK					
Sub Total					
Total					

NUTRIENT	TOTAL	UNITS	GOAL %	RDA%
Calories				
Fat				
Saturated Fat				
Polyunsaturated				
Monounsaturated				

FOOD	QTY	CALS	CARBS	PROTEIN (g)	FAT (g)
BREAKFAST					
Sub Total					
LUNCH					
Sub Total					
DINNER					
Sub Total					
SNACK					
Sub Total					
Total					

NUTRIENT	TOTAL	UNITS	GOAL %	RDA%
Calories				
Fat				
Saturated Fat				
Polyunsaturated				
Monounsaturated				

FOOD	QTY	CALS	CARBS	PROTEIN (g)	FAT (g)
BREAKFAST					
Sub Total					
LUNCH					
Sub Total					
DINNER					
Sub Total					
SNACK					
Sub Total					
Total					

NUTRIENT	TOTAL	UNITS	GOAL %	RDA%
Calories				
Fat				
Saturated Fat				
Polyunsaturated				
Monounsaturated				

FOOD	QTY	CALS	CARBS	PROTEIN (g)	FAT (g)
BREAKFAST					
Sub Total					
LUNCH					
Sub Total					
DINNER					
Sub Total					
SNACK					
Sub Total					
Total					

NUTRIENT	TOTAL	UNITS	GOAL %	RDA%
Calories				
Fat				
Saturated Fat				
Polyunsaturated				
Monounsaturated				

FOOD	QTY	CALS	CARBS	PROTEIN (g)	FAT (g)
BREAKFAST					
Sub Total					
LUNCH					
Sub Total					
DINNER					
Sub Total					
SNACK					
Sub Total					
Total					

NUTRIENT	TOTAL	UNITS	GOAL %	RDA%
Calories				
Fat				
Saturated Fat				
Polyunsaturated				
Monounsaturated				

FOOD	QTY	CALS	CARBS	PROTEIN (g)	FAT (g)
BREAKFAST					
Sub Total					
LUNCH					
Sub Total					
DINNER					
Sub Total					
SNACK					
Sub Total					
Total					

NUTRIENT	TOTAL	UNITS	GOAL %	RDA%
Calories				
Fat				
Saturated Fat				
Polyunsaturated				
Monounsaturated				

FOOD	QTY	CALS	CARBS	PROTEIN (g)	FAT (g)
BREAKFAST					
Sub Total					
LUNCH					
Sub Total					
DINNER					
Sub Total					
SNACK					
Sub Total					
Total					

NUTRIENT	TOTAL	UNITS	GOAL %	RDA%
Calories				
Fat				
Saturated Fat				
Polyunsaturated				
Monounsaturated				

FOOD	QTY	CALS	CARBS	PROTEIN (g)	FAT (g)
BREAKFAST					
Sub Total					
LUNCH					
Sub Total					
DINNER					
Sub Total					
SNACK					
Sub Total					
Total					

NUTRIENT	TOTAL	UNITS	GOAL %	RDA%
Calories				
Fat				
Saturated Fat				
Polyunsaturated				
Monounsaturated				

FOOD	QTY	CALS	CARBS	PROTEIN (g)	FAT (g)
BREAKFAST					
Sub Total					
LUNCH					
Sub Total					
DINNER					
Sub Total					
SNACK					
Sub Total					
Total					

NUTRIENT	TOTAL	UNITS	GOAL %	RDA%
Calories				
Fat				
Saturated Fat				
Polyunsaturated				
Monounsaturated				

FOOD	QTY	CALS	CARBS	PROTEIN (g)	FAT (g)
BREAKFAST					
Sub Total					
LUNCH					
Sub Total					
DINNER					
Sub Total					
SNACK					
Sub Total					
Total					

NUTRIENT	TOTAL	UNITS	GOAL %	RDA%
Calories				
Fat				
Saturated Fat				
Polyunsaturated				
Monounsaturated				

FOOD	QTY	CALS	CARBS	PROTEIN (g)	FAT (g)
BREAKFAST					
Sub Total					
LUNCH					
Sub Total					
DINNER					
Sub Total					
SNACK					
Sub Total					
Total					

NUTRIENT	TOTAL	UNITS	GOAL %	RDA%
Calories				
Fat				
Saturated Fat				
Polyunsaturated				
Monounsaturated				

FOOD	QTY	CALS	CARBS	PROTEIN (g)	FAT (g)
BREAKFAST					
Sub Total					
LUNCH					
Sub Total					
DINNER					
Sub Total					
SNACK					
Sub Total					
Total					

NUTRIENT	TOTAL	UNITS	GOAL %	RDA%
Calories				
Fat				
Saturated Fat				
Polyunsaturated				
Monounsaturated				

FOOD	QTY	CALS	CARBS	PROTEIN (g)	FAT (g)
BREAKFAST					
Sub Total					
LUNCH					
Sub Total					
DINNER					
Sub Total					
SNACK					
Sub Total					
Total					

NUTRIENT	TOTAL	UNITS	GOAL %	RDA%
Calories				
Fat				
Saturated Fat				
Polyunsaturated				
Monounsaturated				

FOOD	QTY	CALS	CARBS	PROTEIN (g)	FAT (g)
BREAKFAST					
Sub Total					
LUNCH					
Sub Total					
DINNER					
Sub Total					
SNACK					
Sub Total					
Total					

NUTRIENT	TOTAL	UNITS	GOAL %	RDA%
Calories				
Fat				
Saturated Fat				
Polyunsaturated				
Monounsaturated				

FOOD	QTY	CALS	CARBS	PROTEIN (g)	FAT (g)
BREAKFAST					
Sub Total					
LUNCH					
Sub Total					
DINNER					
Sub Total					
SNACK					
Sub Total					
Total					

NUTRIENT	TOTAL	UNITS	GOAL %	RDA%
Calories				
Fat				
Saturated Fat				
Polyunsaturated				
Monounsaturated				

FOOD	QTY	CALS	CARBS	PROTEIN (g)	FAT (g)
BREAKFAST					
Sub Total					
LUNCH					
Sub Total					
DINNER					
Sub Total					
SNACK					
Sub Total					
Total					

NUTRIENT	TOTAL	UNITS	GOAL %	RDA%
Calories				
Fat				
Saturated Fat				
Polyunsaturated				
Monounsaturated				

FOOD	QTY	CALS	CARBS	PROTEIN (g)	FAT (g)
BREAKFAST					
Sub Total					
LUNCH					
Sub Total					
DINNER					
Sub Total					
SNACK					
Sub Total					
Total					

NUTRIENT	TOTAL	UNITS	GOAL %	RDA%
Calories				
Fat				
Saturated Fat				
Polyunsaturated				
Monounsaturated				

FOOD	QTY	CALS	CARBS	PROTEIN (g)	FAT (g)
BREAKFAST					
Sub Total					
LUNCH					
Sub Total					
DINNER					
Sub Total					
SNACK					
Sub Total					
Total					

NUTRIENT	TOTAL	UNITS	GOAL %	RDA%
Calories				
Fat				
Saturated Fat				
Polyunsaturated				
Monounsaturated				

FOOD	QTY	CALS	CARBS	PROTEIN (g)	FAT (g)
BREAKFAST					
Sub Total					
LUNCH					
Sub Total					
DINNER					
Sub Total					
SNACK					
Sub Total					
Total					

NUTRIENT	TOTAL	UNITS	GOAL %	RDA%
Calories				
Fat				
Saturated Fat				
Polyunsaturated				
Monounsaturated				

FOOD	QTY	CALS	CARBS	PROTEIN (g)	FAT (g)
BREAKFAST					
Sub Total					
LUNCH					
Sub Total					
DINNER					
Sub Total					
SNACK					
Sub Total					
Total					

NUTRIENT	TOTAL	UNITS	GOAL %	RDA%
Calories				
Fat				
Saturated Fat				
Polyunsaturated				
Monounsaturated				

FOOD	QTY	CALS	CARBS	PROTEIN (g)	FAT (g)
BREAKFAST					
Sub Total					
LUNCH					
Sub Total					
DINNER					
Sub Total					
SNACK					
Sub Total					
Total					

NUTRIENT	TOTAL	UNITS	GOAL %	RDA%
Calories				
Fat				
Saturated Fat				
Polyunsaturated				
Monounsaturated				

FOOD	QTY	CALS	CARBS	PROTEIN (g)	FAT (g)
BREAKFAST					
Sub Total					
LUNCH					
Sub Total					
DINNER					
Sub Total					
SNACK					
Sub Total					
Total					

NUTRIENT	TOTAL	UNITS	GOAL %	RDA%
Calories				
Fat				
Saturated Fat				
Polyunsaturated				
Monounsaturated				

FOOD	QTY	CALS	CARBS	PROTEIN (g)	FAT (g)
BREAKFAST					
Sub Total					
LUNCH					
Sub Total					
DINNER					
Sub Total					
SNACK					
Sub Total					
Total					

NUTRIENT	TOTAL	UNITS	GOAL %	RDA%
Calories				
Fat				
Saturated Fat				
Polyunsaturated				
Monounsaturated				

FOOD		QTY	CALS	CARBS	PROTEIN (g)	FAT (g)
BREAKFAST						
	Sub Total					
LUNCH						
	Sub Total					
DINNER						
	Sub Total					
SNACK						
	Sub Total					
	Total					

NUTRIENT	TOTAL	UNITS	GOAL %	RDA%
Calories				
Fat				
Saturated Fat				
Polyunsaturated				
Monounsaturated				

FOOD	QTY	CALS	CARBS	PROTEIN (g)	FAT (g)
BREAKFAST					
Sub Total					
LUNCH					
Sub Total					
DINNER					
Sub Total					
SNACK					
Sub Total					
Total					

NUTRIENT	TOTAL	UNITS	GOAL %	RDA%
Calories				
Fat				
Saturated Fat				
Polyunsaturated				
Monounsaturated				

FOOD	QTY	CALS	CARBS	PROTEIN (g)	FAT (g)
BREAKFAST					
Sub Total					
LUNCH					
Sub Total					
DINNER					
Sub Total					
SNACK					
Sub Total					
Total					

NUTRIENT	TOTAL	UNITS	GOAL %	RDA%
Calories				
Fat				
Saturated Fat				
Polyunsaturated				
Monounsaturated				

FOOD	QTY	CALS	CARBS	PROTEIN (g)	FAT (g)
BREAKFAST					
Sub Total					
LUNCH					
Sub Total					
DINNER					
Sub Total					
SNACK					
Sub Total					
Total					

NUTRIENT	TOTAL	UNITS	GOAL %	RDA%
Calories				
Fat				
Saturated Fat				
Polyunsaturated				
Monounsaturated				

FOOD	QTY	CALS	CARBS	PROTEIN (g)	FAT (g)
BREAKFAST					
Sub Total					
LUNCH					
Sub Total					
DINNER					
Sub Total					
SNACK					
Sub Total					
Total					

NUTRIENT	TOTAL	UNITS	GOAL %	RDA%
Calories				
Fat				
Saturated Fat				
Polyunsaturated				
Monounsaturated				

FOOD	QTY	CALS	CARBS	PROTEIN (g)	FAT (g)
BREAKFAST					
Sub Total					
LUNCH					
Sub Total					
DINNER					
Sub Total					
SNACK					
Sub Total					
Total					

NUTRIENT	TOTAL	UNITS	GOAL %	RDA%
Calories				
Fat				
Saturated Fat				
Polyunsaturated				
Monounsaturated				

FOOD	QTY	CALS	CARBS	PROTEIN (g)	FAT (g)
BREAKFAST					
Sub Total					
LUNCH					
Sub Total					
DINNER					
Sub Total					
SNACK					
Sub Total					
Total					

NUTRIENT	TOTAL	UNITS	GOAL %	RDA%
Calories				
Fat				
Saturated Fat				
Polyunsaturated				
Monounsaturated				

FOOD	QTY	CALS	CARBS	PROTEIN (g)	FAT (g)
BREAKFAST					
Sub Total					
LUNCH					
Sub Total					
DINNER					
Sub Total					
SNACK					
Sub Total					
Total					

NUTRIENT	TOTAL	UNITS	GOAL %	RDA%
Calories				
Fat				
Saturated Fat				
Polyunsaturated				
Monounsaturated				

FOOD		QTY	CALS	CARBS	PROTEIN (g)	FAT (g)
BREAKFAST						
	Sub Total					
LUNCH						
	Sub Total					
DINNER						
	Sub Total					
SNACK						
	Sub Total					
	Total					

NUTRIENT	TOTAL	UNITS	GOAL %	RDA%
Calories				
Fat				
Saturated Fat				
Polyunsaturated				
Monounsaturated				

FOOD	QTY	CALS	CARBS	PROTEIN (g)	FAT (g)
BREAKFAST					
Sub Total					
LUNCH					
Sub Total					
DINNER					
Sub Total					
SNACK					
Sub Total					
Total					

NUTRIENT	TOTAL	UNITS	GOAL %	RDA%
Calories				
Fat				
Saturated Fat				
Polyunsaturated				
Monounsaturated				

FOOD	QTY	CALS	CARBS	PROTEIN (g)	FAT (g)
BREAKFAST					
Sub Total					
LUNCH					
Sub Total					
DINNER					
Sub Total					
SNACK					
Sub Total					
Total					

NUTRIENT	TOTAL	UNITS	GOAL %	RDA%
Calories				
Fat				
Saturated Fat				
Polyunsaturated				
Monounsaturated				

FOOD	QTY	CALS	CARBS	PROTEIN (g)	FAT (g)
BREAKFAST					
Sub Total					
LUNCH					
Sub Total					
DINNER					
Sub Total					
SNACK					
Sub Total					
Total					

NUTRIENT	TOTAL	UNITS	GOAL %	RDA%
Calories				
Fat				
Saturated Fat				
Polyunsaturated				
Monounsaturated				

FOOD	QTY	CALS	CARBS	PROTEIN (g)	FAT (g)
BREAKFAST					
Sub Total					
LUNCH					
Sub Total					
DINNER					
Sub Total					
SNACK					
Sub Total					
Total					

NUTRIENT	TOTAL	UNITS	GOAL %	RDA%
Calories				
Fat				
Saturated Fat				
Polyunsaturated				
Monounsaturated				

FOOD	QTY	CALS	CARBS	PROTEIN (g)	FAT (g)
BREAKFAST					
Sub Total					
LUNCH					
Sub Total					
DINNER					
Sub Total					
SNACK					
Sub Total					
Total					

NUTRIENT	TOTAL	UNITS	GOAL %	RDA%
Calories				
Fat				
Saturated Fat				
Polyunsaturated				
Monounsaturated				

FOOD	QTY	CALS	CARBS	PROTEIN (g)	FAT (g)
BREAKFAST					
Sub Total					
LUNCH					
Sub Total					
DINNER					
Sub Total					
SNACK					
Sub Total					
Total					

NUTRIENT	TOTAL	UNITS	GOAL %	RDA%
Calories				
Fat				
Saturated Fat				
Polyunsaturated				
Monounsaturated				

FOOD	QTY	CALS	CARBS	PROTEIN (g)	FAT (g)
BREAKFAST					
Sub Total					
LUNCH					
Sub Total					
DINNER					
Sub Total					
SNACK					
Sub Total					
Total					

NUTRIENT	TOTAL	UNITS	GOAL %	RDA%
Calories				
Fat				
Saturated Fat				
Polyunsaturated				
Monounsaturated				

FOOD	QTY	CALS	CARBS	PROTEIN (g)	FAT (g)
BREAKFAST					
Sub Total					
LUNCH					
Sub Total					
DINNER					
Sub Total					
SNACK					
Sub Total					
Total					

NUTRIENT	TOTAL	UNITS	GOAL %	RDA%
Calories				
Fat				
Saturated Fat				
Polyunsaturated				
Monounsaturated				

FOOD	QTY	CALS	CARBS	PROTEIN (g)	FAT (g)
BREAKFAST					
Sub Total					
LUNCH					
Sub Total					
DINNER					
Sub Total					
SNACK					
Sub Total					
Total					

NUTRIENT	TOTAL	UNITS	GOAL %	RDA%
Calories				
Fat				
Saturated Fat				
Polyunsaturated				
Monounsaturated				

FOOD	QTY	CALS	CARBS	PROTEIN (g)	FAT (g)
BREAKFAST					
Sub Total					
LUNCH					
Sub Total					
DINNER					
Sub Total					
SNACK					
Sub Total					
Total					

NUTRIENT	TOTAL	UNITS	GOAL %	RDA%
Calories				
Fat				
Saturated Fat				
Polyunsaturated				
Monounsaturated				

FOOD	QTY	CALS	CARBS	PROTEIN (g)	FAT (g)
BREAKFAST					
Sub Total					
LUNCH					
Sub Total					
DINNER					
Sub Total					
SNACK					
Sub Total					
Total					

NUTRIENT	TOTAL	UNITS	GOAL %	RDA%
Calories				
Fat				
Saturated Fat				
Polyunsaturated				
Monounsaturated				

FOOD	QTY	CALS	CARBS	PROTEIN (g)	FAT (g)
BREAKFAST					
Sub Total					
LUNCH					
Sub Total					
DINNER					
Sub Total					
SNACK					
Sub Total					
Total					

NUTRIENT	TOTAL	UNITS	GOAL %	RDA%
Calories				
Fat				
Saturated Fat				
Polyunsaturated				
Monounsaturated				

FOOD	QTY	CALS	CARBS	PROTEIN (g)	FAT (g)
BREAKFAST					
Sub Total					
LUNCH					
Sub Total					
DINNER					
Sub Total					
SNACK					
Sub Total					
Total					

NUTRIENT	TOTAL	UNITS	GOAL %	RDA%
Calories				
Fat				
Saturated Fat				
Polyunsaturated				
Monounsaturated				

FOOD	QTY	CALS	CARBS	PROTEIN (g)	FAT (g)
BREAKFAST					
Sub Total					
LUNCH					
Sub Total					
DINNER					
Sub Total					
SNACK					
Sub Total					
Total					

NUTRIENT	TOTAL	UNITS	GOAL %	RDA%
Calories				
Fat				
Saturated Fat				
Polyunsaturated				
Monounsaturated				

FOOD	QTY	CALS	CARBS	PROTEIN (g)	FAT (g)
BREAKFAST					
Sub Total					
LUNCH					
Sub Total					
DINNER					
Sub Total					
SNACK					
Sub Total					
Total					

NUTRIENT	TOTAL	UNITS	GOAL %	RDA%
Calories				
Fat				
Saturated Fat				
Polyunsaturated				
Monounsaturated				

FOOD	QTY	CALS	CARBS	PROTEIN (g)	FAT (g)
BREAKFAST					
Sub Total					
LUNCH					
Sub Total					
DINNER					
Sub Total					
SNACK					
Sub Total					
Total					

NUTRIENT	TOTAL	UNITS	GOAL %	RDA%
Calories				
Fat				
Saturated Fat				
Polyunsaturated				
Monounsaturated				

FOOD	QTY	CALS	CARBS	PROTEIN (g)	FAT (g)
BREAKFAST					
Sub Total					
LUNCH					
Sub Total					
DINNER					
Sub Total					
SNACK					
Sub Total					
Total					

NUTRIENT	TOTAL	UNITS	GOAL %	RDA%
Calories				
Fat				
Saturated Fat				
Polyunsaturated				
Monounsaturated				

FOOD	QTY	CALS	CARBS	PROTEIN (g)	FAT (g)
BREAKFAST					
Sub Total					
LUNCH					
Sub Total					
DINNER					
Sub Total					
SNACK					
Sub Total					
Total					

NUTRIENT	TOTAL	UNITS	GOAL %	RDA%
Calories				
Fat				
Saturated Fat				
Polyunsaturated				
Monounsaturated				

FOOD	QTY	CALS	CARBS	PROTEIN (g)	FAT (g)
BREAKFAST					
Sub Total					
LUNCH					
Sub Total					
DINNER					
Sub Total					
SNACK					
Sub Total					
Total					

NUTRIENT	TOTAL	UNITS	GOAL %	RDA%
Calories				
Fat				
Saturated Fat				
Polyunsaturated				
Monounsaturated				

FOOD	QTY	CALS	CARBS	PROTEIN (g)	FAT (g)
BREAKFAST					
Sub Total					
LUNCH					
Sub Total					
DINNER					
Sub Total					
SNACK					
Sub Total					
Total					

NUTRIENT	TOTAL	UNITS	GOAL %	RDA%
Calories				
Fat				
Saturated Fat				
Polyunsaturated				
Monounsaturated				

FOOD	QTY	CALS	CARBS	PROTEIN (g)	FAT (g)
BREAKFAST					
Sub Total					
LUNCH					
Sub Total					
DINNER					
Sub Total					
SNACK					
Sub Total					
Total					

NUTRIENT	TOTAL	UNITS	GOAL %	RDA%
Calories				
Fat				
Saturated Fat				
Polyunsaturated				
Monounsaturated				

FOOD	QTY	CALS	CARBS	PROTEIN (g)	FAT (g)
BREAKFAST					
Sub Total					
LUNCH					
Sub Total					
DINNER					
Sub Total					
SNACK					
Sub Total					
Total					

NUTRIENT	TOTAL	UNITS	GOAL %	RDA%
Calories				
Fat				
Saturated Fat				
Polyunsaturated				
Monounsaturated				

FOOD	QTY	CALS	CARBS	PROTEIN (g)	FAT (g)
BREAKFAST					
Sub Total					
LUNCH					
Sub Total					
DINNER					
Sub Total					
SNACK					
Sub Total					
Total					

NUTRIENT	TOTAL	UNITS	GOAL %	RDA%
Calories				
Fat				
Saturated Fat				
Polyunsaturated				
Monounsaturated				

FOOD	QTY	CALS	CARBS	PROTEIN (g)	FAT (g)
BREAKFAST					
Sub Total					
LUNCH					
Sub Total					
DINNER					
Sub Total					
SNACK					
Sub Total					
Total					

NUTRIENT	TOTAL	UNITS	GOAL %	RDA%
Calories				
Fat				
Saturated Fat				
Polyunsaturated				
Monounsaturated				

FOOD	QTY	CALS	CARBS	PROTEIN (g)	FAT (g)
BREAKFAST					
Sub Total					
LUNCH					
Sub Total					
DINNER					
Sub Total					
SNACK					
Sub Total					
Total					

NUTRIENT	TOTAL	UNITS	GOAL %	RDA%
Calories				
Fat				
Saturated Fat				
Polyunsaturated				
Monounsaturated				

FOOD	QTY	CALS	CARBS	PROTEIN (g)	FAT (g)
BREAKFAST					
Sub Total					
LUNCH					
Sub Total					
DINNER					
Sub Total					
SNACK					
Sub Total					
Total					

NUTRIENT	TOTAL	UNITS	GOAL %	RDA%
Calories				
Fat				
Saturated Fat				
Polyunsaturated				
Monounsaturated				

FOOD	QTY	CALS	CARBS	PROTEIN (g)	FAT (g)
BREAKFAST					
Sub Total					
LUNCH					
Sub Total					
DINNER					
Sub Total					
SNACK					
Sub Total					
Total					

NUTRIENT	TOTAL	UNITS	GOAL %	RDA%
Calories				
Fat				
Saturated Fat				
Polyunsaturated				
Monounsaturated				

FOOD		QTY	CALS	CARBS	PROTEIN (g)	FAT (g)
BREAKFAST						
	Sub Total					
LUNCH						
	Sub Total					
DINNER						
	Sub Total					
SNACK						
	Sub Total					
	Total					

NUTRIENT	TOTAL	UNITS	GOAL %	RDA%
Calories				
Fat				
Saturated Fat				
Polyunsaturated				
Monounsaturated				

FOOD	QTY	CALS	CARBS	PROTEIN (g)	FAT (g)
BREAKFAST					
Sub Total					
LUNCH					
Sub Total					
DINNER					
Sub Total					
SNACK					
Sub Total					
Total					

NUTRIENT	TOTAL	UNITS	GOAL %	RDA%
Calories				
Fat				
Saturated Fat				
Polyunsaturated				
Monounsaturated				

FOOD	QTY	CALS	CARBS	PROTEIN (g)	FAT (g)
BREAKFAST					
Sub Total					
LUNCH					
Sub Total					
DINNER					
Sub Total					
SNACK					
Sub Total					
Total					

NUTRIENT	TOTAL	UNITS	GOAL %	RDA%
Calories				
Fat				
Saturated Fat				
Polyunsaturated				
Monounsaturated				

FOOD	QTY	CALS	CARBS	PROTEIN (g)	FAT (g)
BREAKFAST					
Sub Total					
LUNCH					
Sub Total					
DINNER					
Sub Total					
SNACK					
Sub Total					
Total					

NUTRIENT	TOTAL	UNITS	GOAL %	RDA%
Calories				
Fat				
Saturated Fat				
Polyunsaturated				
Monounsaturated				

FOOD		QTY	CALS	CARBS	PROTEIN (g)	FAT (g)
BREAKFAST						
	Sub Total					
LUNCH						
	Sub Total					
DINNER						
	Sub Total					
SNACK						
	Sub Total					
	Total					

NUTRIENT	TOTAL	UNITS	GOAL %	RDA%
Calories				
Fat				
Saturated Fat				
Polyunsaturated				
Monounsaturated				

FOOD	QTY	CALS	CARBS	PROTEIN (g)	FAT (g)
BREAKFAST					
Sub Total					
LUNCH					
Sub Total					
DINNER					
Sub Total					
SNACK					
Sub Total					
Total					

NUTRIENT	TOTAL	UNITS	GOAL %	RDA%
Calories				
Fat				
Saturated Fat				
Polyunsaturated				
Monounsaturated				

FOOD	QTY	CALS	CARBS	PROTEIN (g)	FAT (g)
BREAKFAST					
Sub Total					
LUNCH					
Sub Total					
DINNER					
Sub Total					
SNACK					
Sub Total					
Total					

NUTRIENT	TOTAL	UNITS	GOAL %	RDA%
Calories				
Fat				
Saturated Fat				
Polyunsaturated				
Monounsaturated				

FOOD	QTY	CALS	CARBS	PROTEIN (g)	FAT (g)
BREAKFAST					
Sub Total					
LUNCH					
Sub Total					
DINNER					
Sub Total					
SNACK					
Sub Total					
Total					

NUTRIENT	TOTAL	UNITS	GOAL %	RDA%
Calories				
Fat				
Saturated Fat				
Polyunsaturated				
Monounsaturated				